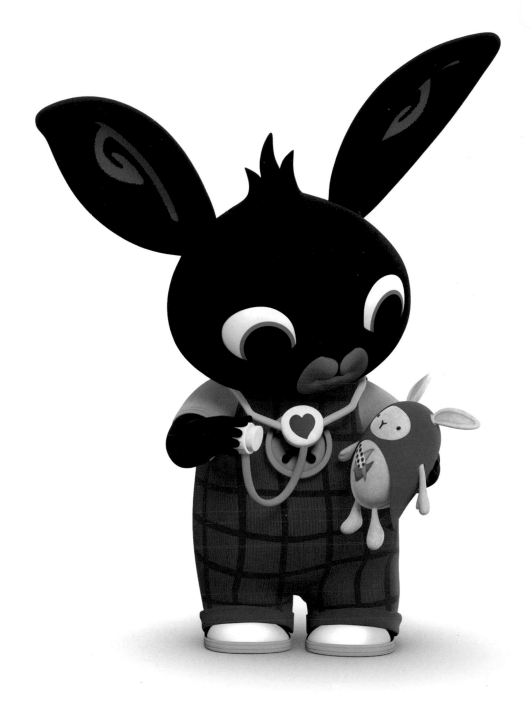

This Bing book belongs to

. . . .

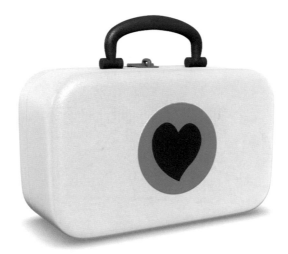

The *Bing* television series is created by Acamar Films and Brown Bag Films
and adapted from the original books by Ted Dewan.

Doctor Bing is based on the original story *Vaccination* written by Denise Cassar, Mikael Shields and Claire Jennings.
Doctor Bing was first published in Great Britain by HarperCollins *Children's Books* in 2021
and was adapted from the original story by Lauren Holowaty.

HarperCollins *Children's Books* is a division of HarperCollins*Publishers* Ltd,
1 London Bridge Street, London SE1 9GF

www.harpercollins.co.uk

HarperCollins*Publishers*
1st Floor, Watermarque Building, Ringsend Road, Dublin 4, Ireland

1 3 5 7 9 10 8 6 4 2

ISBN: 978-0-00-847563-5

Printed in Poland

MIX
Paper from
responsible sources
FSC
www.fsc.org   FSC® C007454

This book is produced from independently certified FSC™ paper
to ensure responsible forest management.

For more information visit: www.harpercollins.co.uk/green

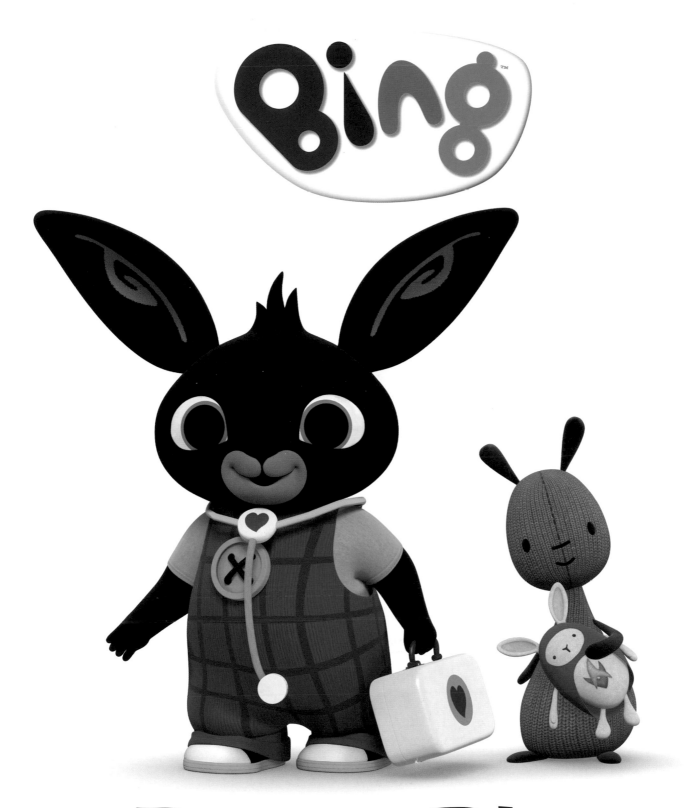

Doctor Bing

HarperCollins *Children's Books*

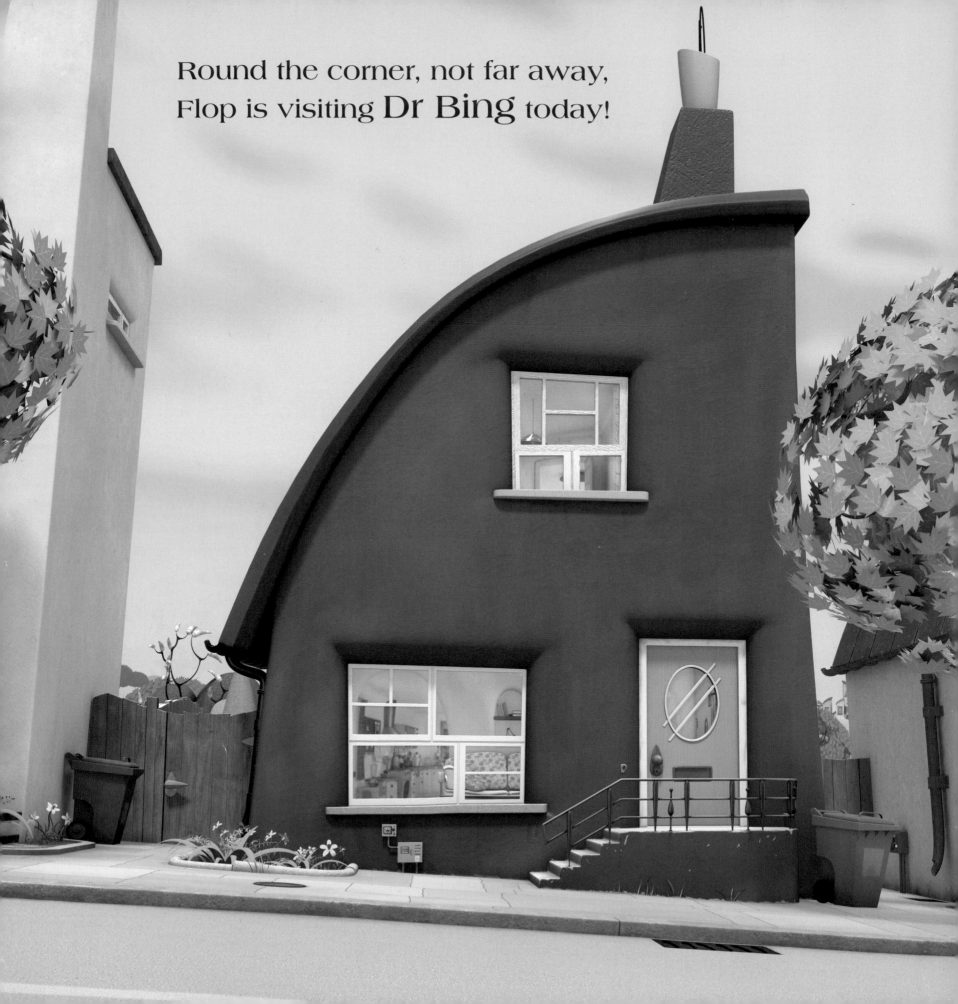

Round the corner, not far away,
Flop is visiting **Dr Bing** today!

Flop taps on the table.

Knock, knock!

"Yes," answers Bing. "Come in!"

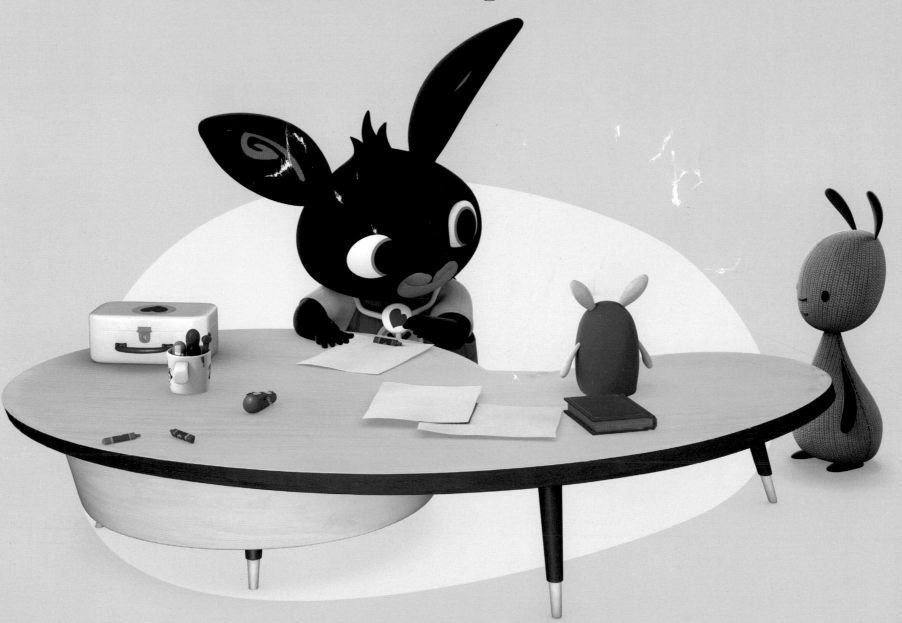

"Morning, Dr Bing," says Flop.
"Sit down and I'll do your vaccination,"
says Dr Bing, pointing to the sofa.

Dr Bing explains to Flop what a vaccination is.
"It's medicine for the inside of your body – so you
don't get sick. It's just a teeny-tiny scratch . . .

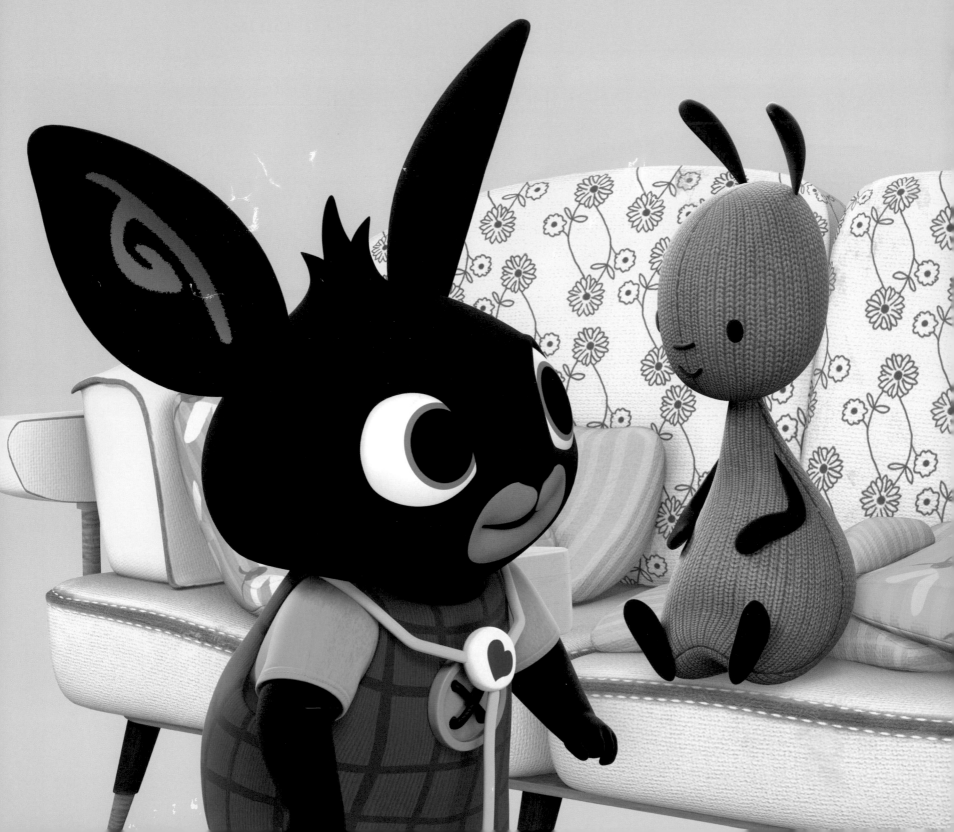

and after, you'll get a special... shiny... Hoppity Voosh Sticker!" says Bing, "Ready?"
"I think so," replies Flop.
"All done!" announces Dr Bing.
"Oh, that didn't hurt as much as I thought," says Flop.

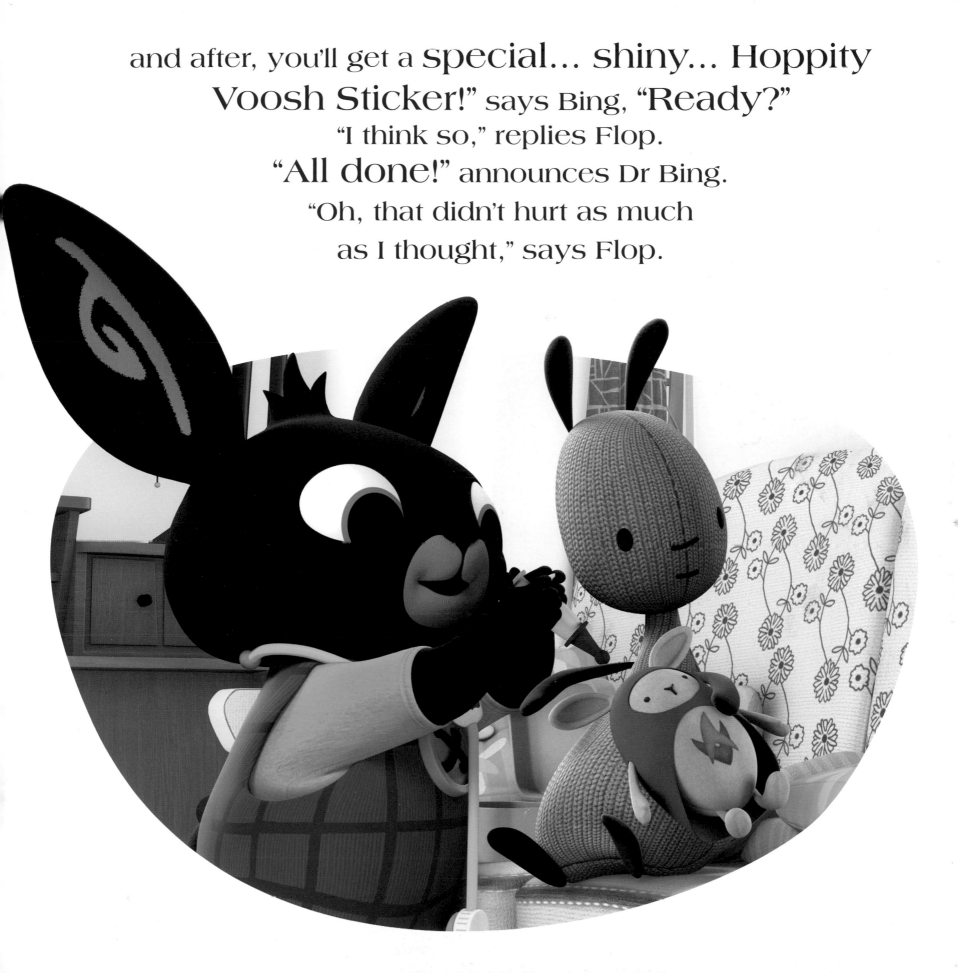

Flop tells Bing that it's time to go to
Dr Molly's clinic for *his* vaccination now.

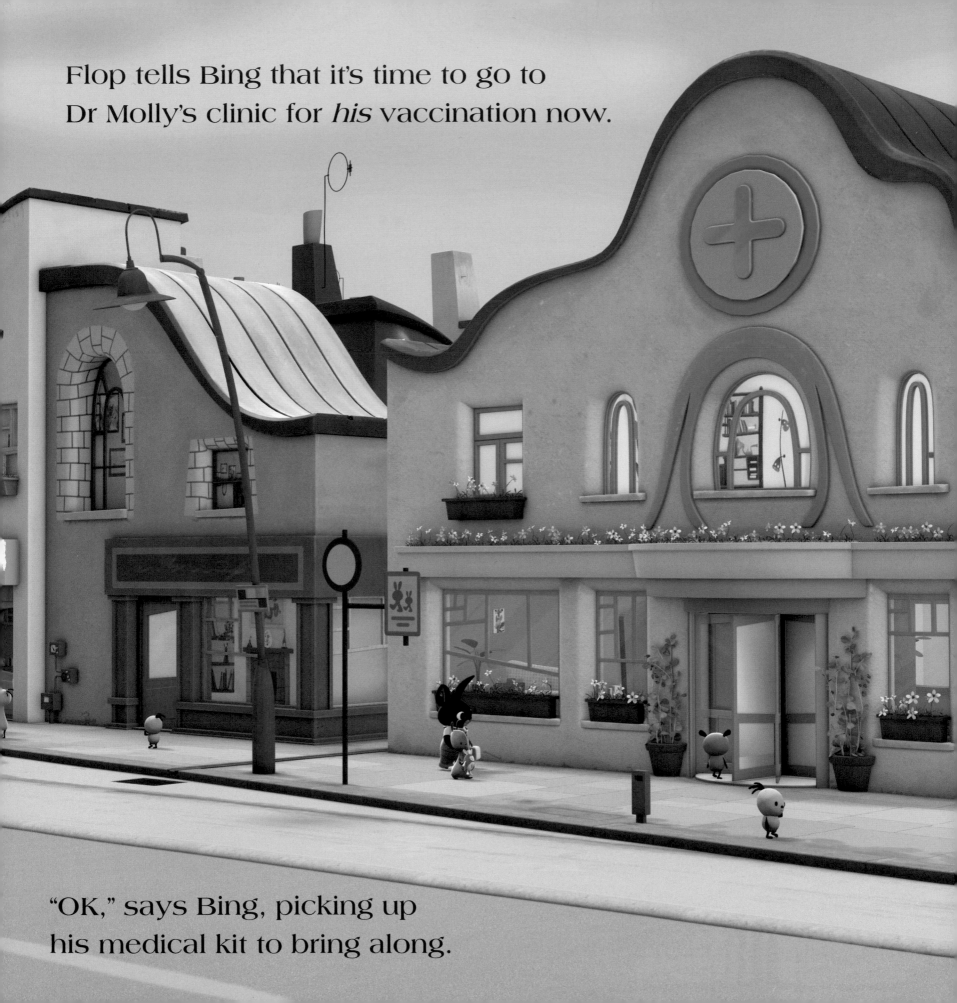

"OK," says Bing, picking up
his medical kit to bring along.

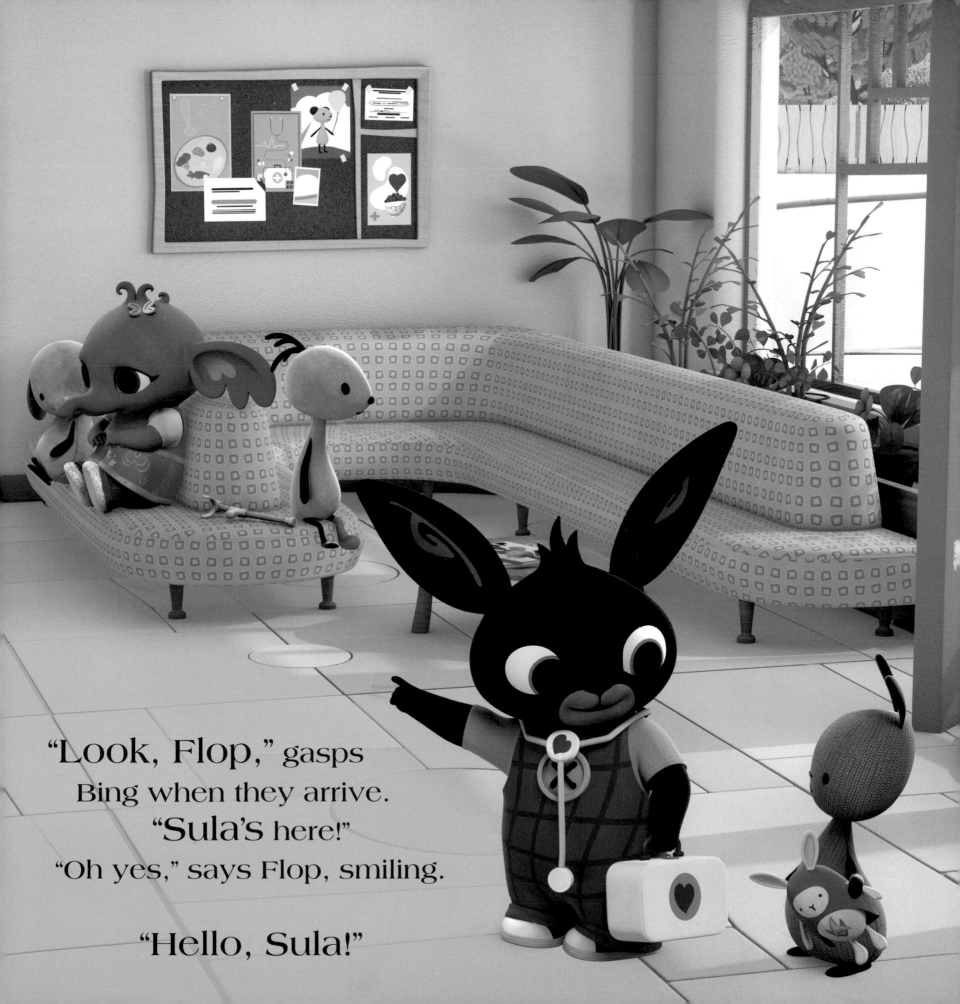

"Look, Flop," gasps
Bing when they arrive.
"Sula's here!"
"Oh yes," says Flop, smiling.

"Hello, Sula!"

"I'm having my vaccination,"
Bing tells Sula proudly.
"Me too," Sula says softly.

Dr Molly comes out
of her office. "Hello,
Sula. Hello, Bing."

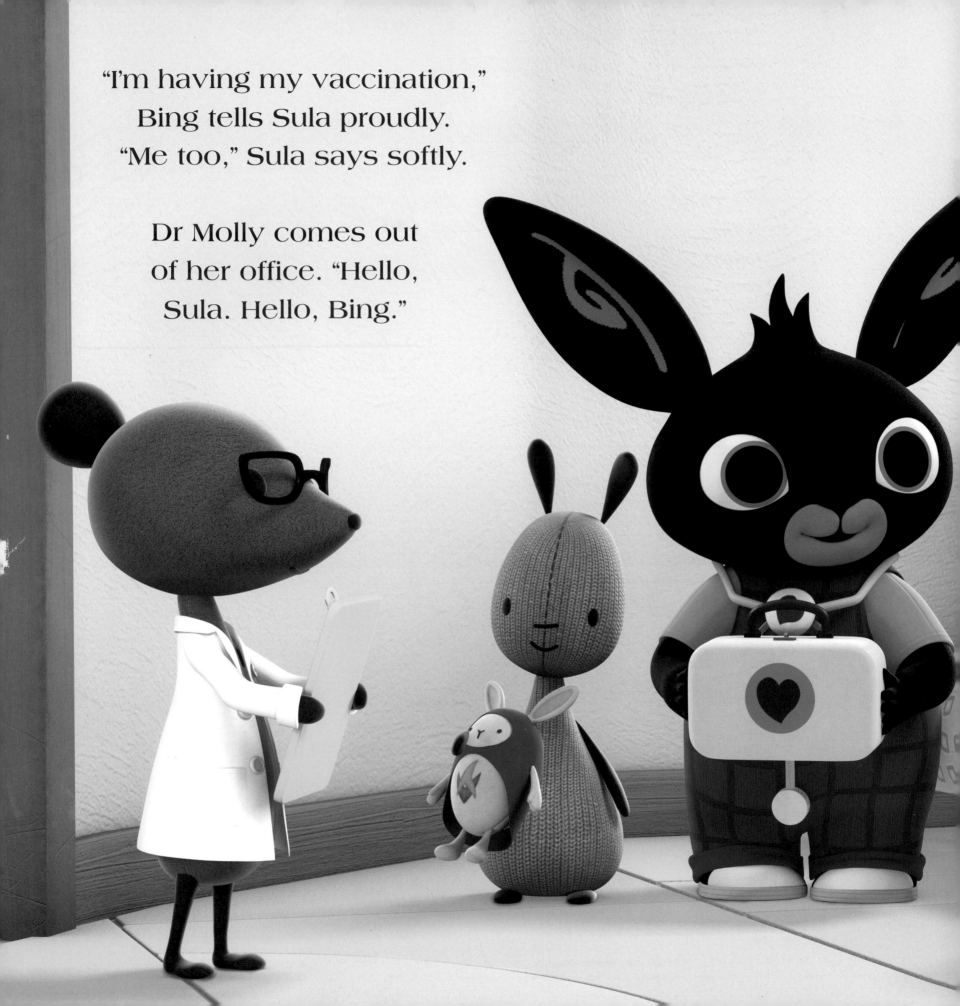

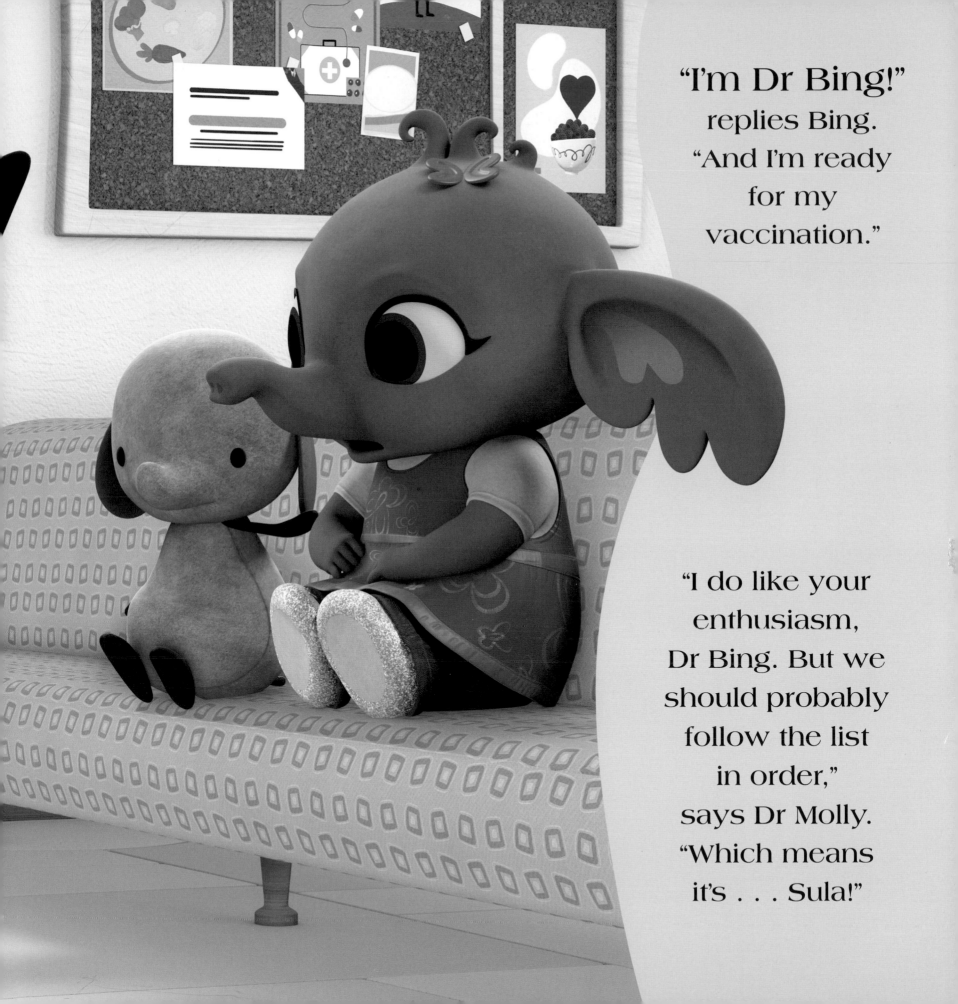

"I'm Dr Bing!" replies Bing. "And I'm ready for my vaccination."

"I do like your enthusiasm, Dr Bing. But we should probably follow the list in order," says Dr Molly. "Which means it's . . . Sula!"

Sula is a **bit nervous**. "I don't want my vaccination," she says quietly.

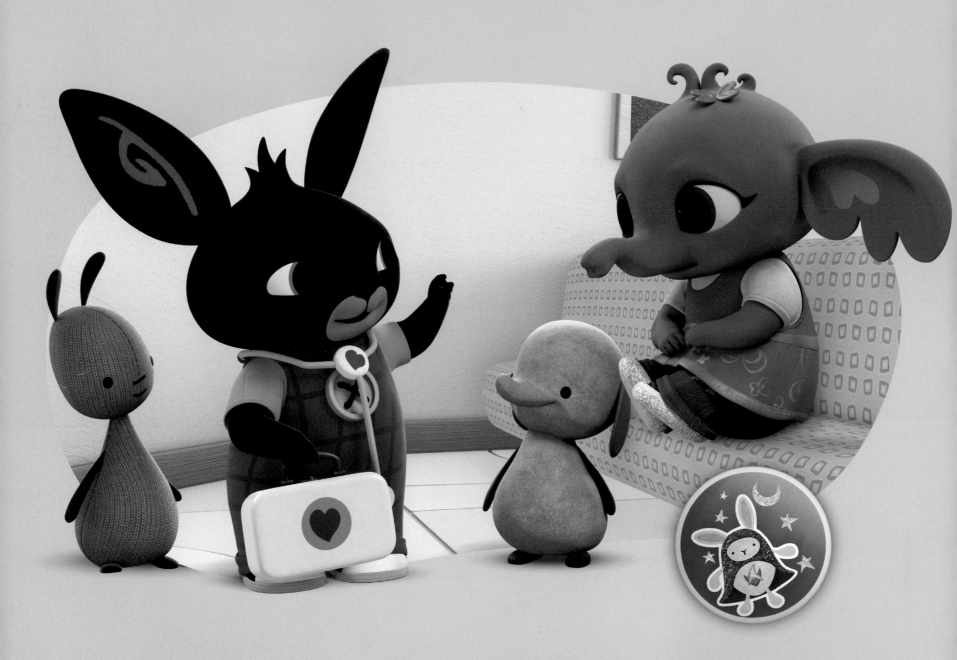

"Don't worry, Sula," says Bing. "There's a teeny-tiny scratch but then you get a special . . . shiny. . . Hoppity Voosh sticker!"

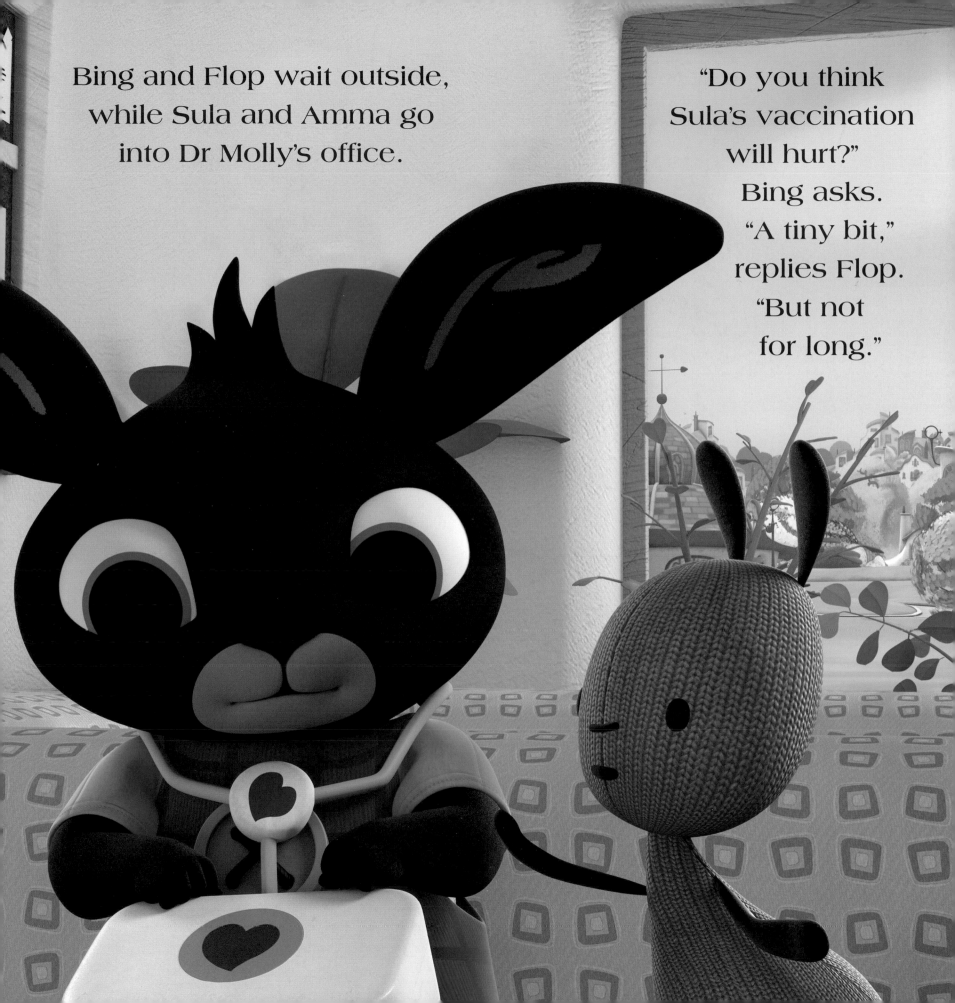

Bing and Flop wait outside,
while Sula and Amma go
into Dr Molly's office.

"Do you think
Sula's vaccination
will hurt?"
Bing asks.
"A tiny bit,"
replies Flop.
"But not
for long."

Sula walks out
of Dr Molly's
office smiling.
"Look!"
she gasps.

"I got a Hoppity
Voosh sticker!"
"Ohhh . . .YES!"
gasps Bing,
hopping off the chair.
"Well done, Sula,"
says Flop.

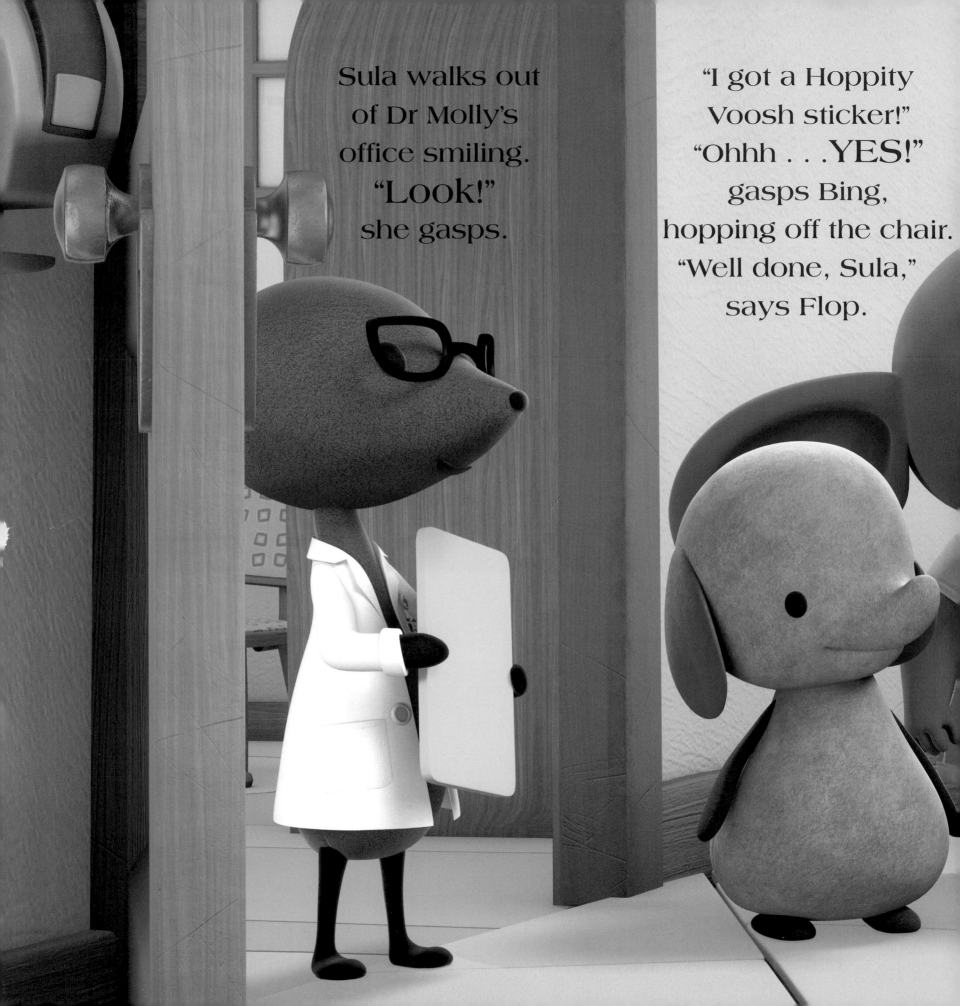

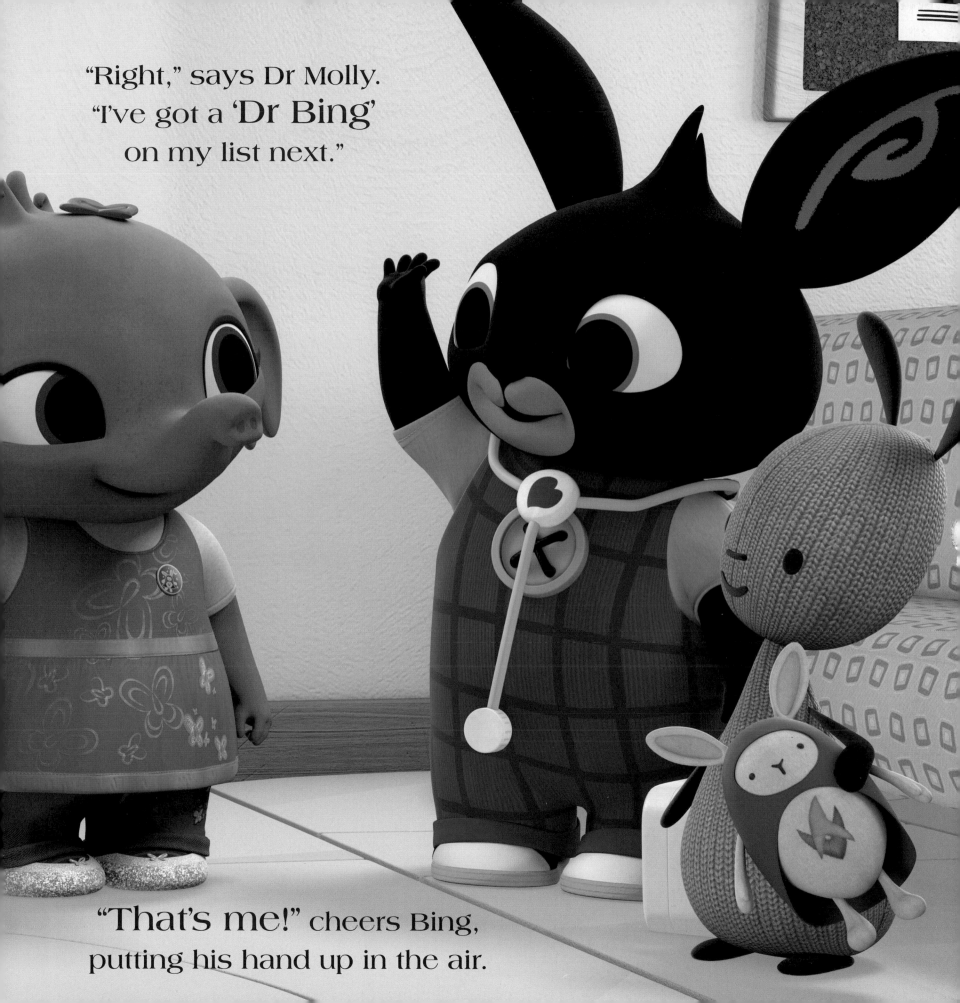

"Right," says Dr Molly. "I've got a 'Dr Bing' on my list next."

"That's me!" cheers Bing, putting his hand up in the air.

Dr Molly rolls up Bing's sleeve and he shuts his eyes.
And with one tiny little scratch the vaccination is done.
"Ohh, um... it didn't hurt hardly at all," says Bing.
"Good for you, Bing," says Flop.

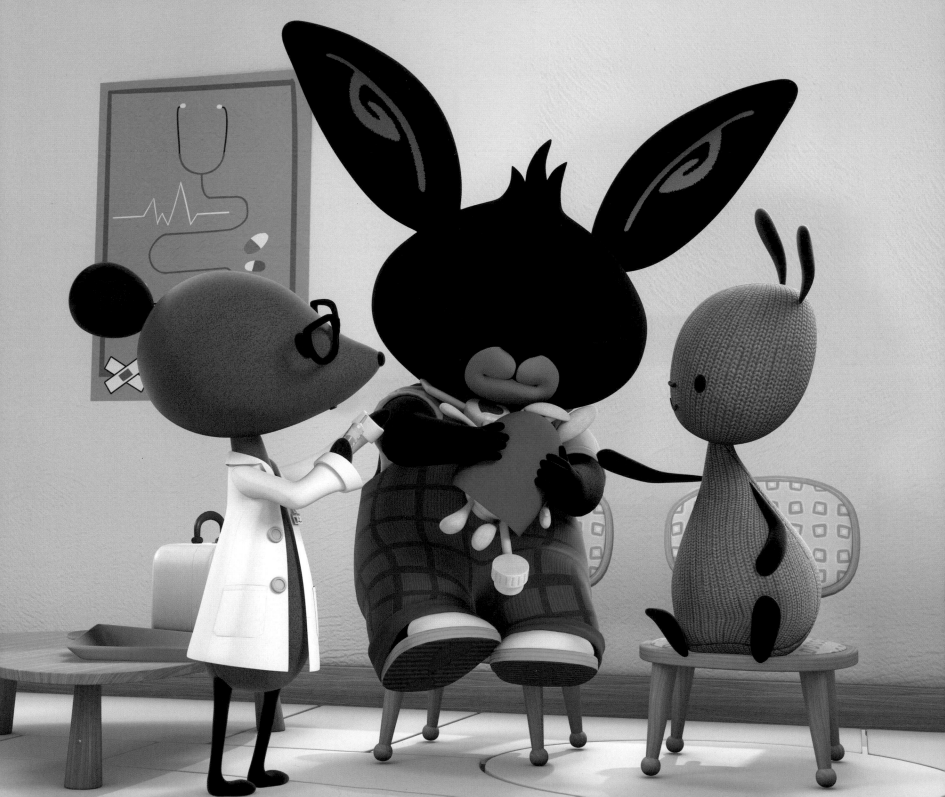

"Um . . . could I have a shiny Hoppity Voosh sticker, please?" asks Bing.

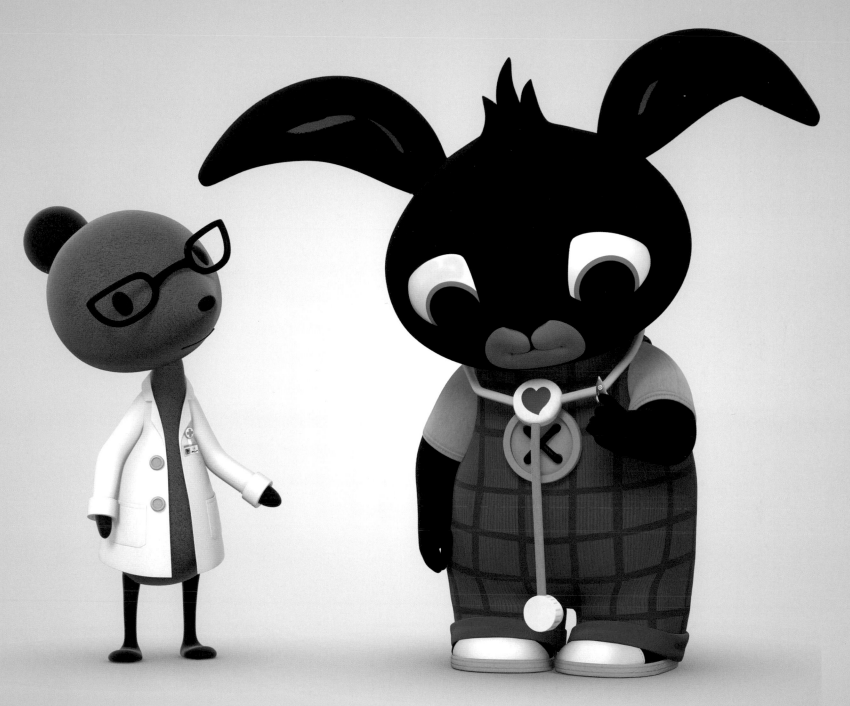

"Oh gosh, I don't have any more of those," says Dr Molly.
She gives Bing a smiley-face rocket sticker instead.
"Thank you," says Bing sadly.

On his way out, Bing walks past
Pando. Bing looks sad because
he is disappointed he didn't get his
special shiny Hoppity Voosh sticker.

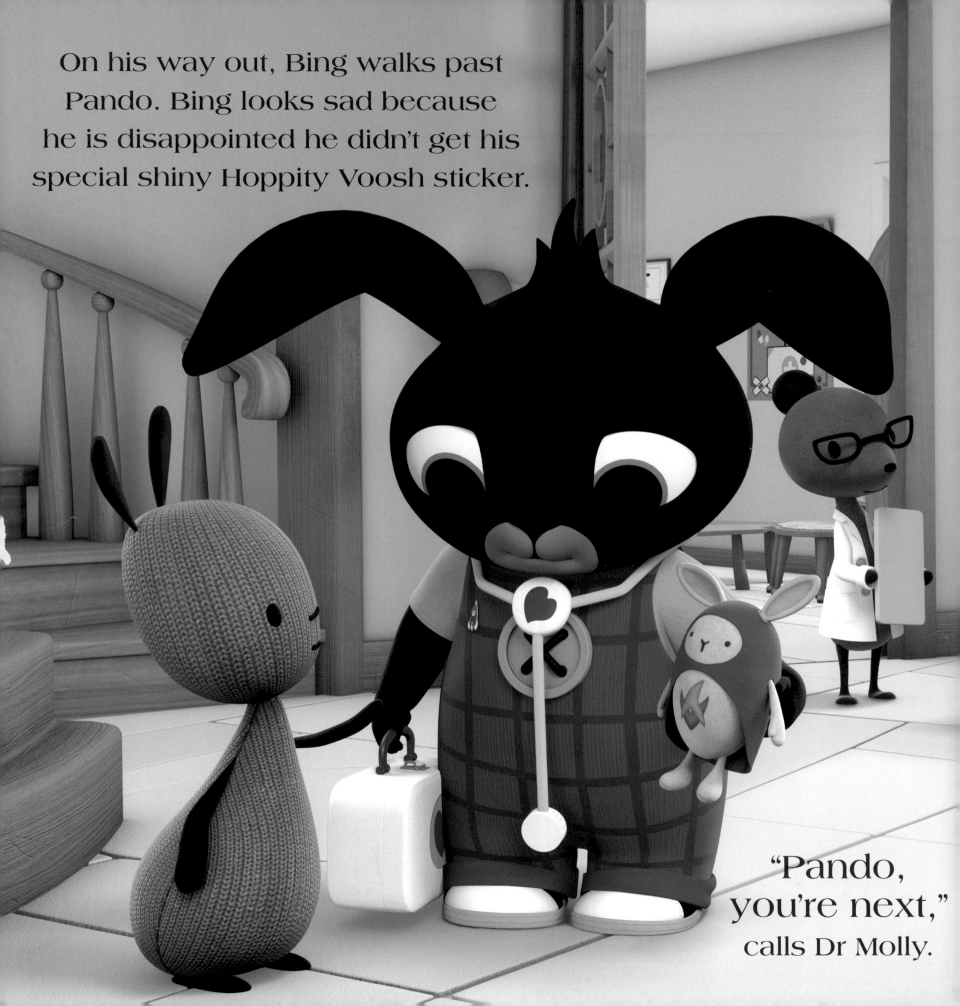

"Pando,
you're next,"
calls Dr Molly.

"I don't want my vaccination!"
says Pando, seeing Bing's upset face.
"It'll hurt like Bing's did."

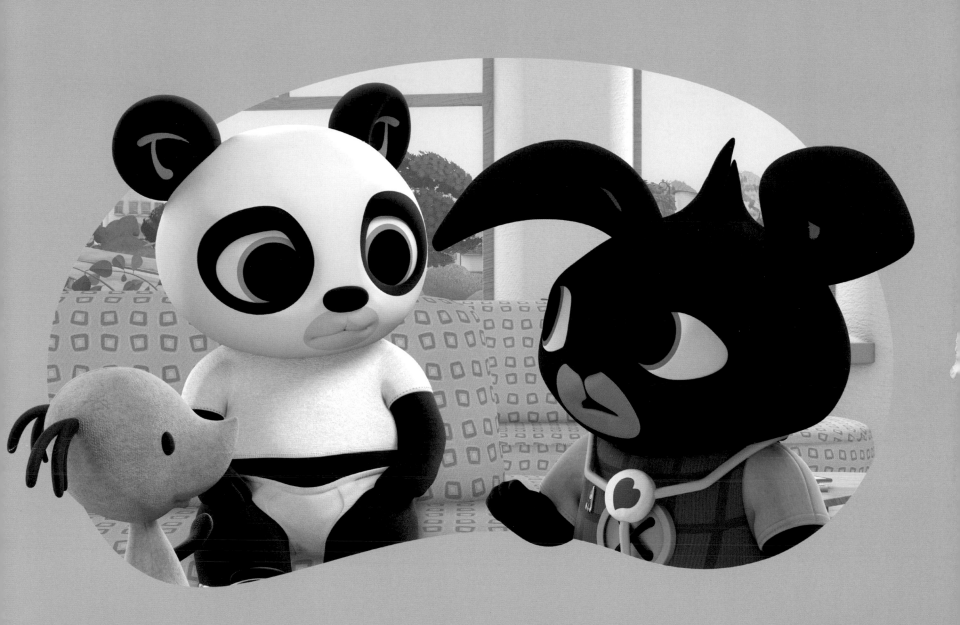

"Mine didn't hurt hardly at all," explains
Dr Bing. "I'm upset because I didn't get
a special shiny Hoppity Voosh sticker."

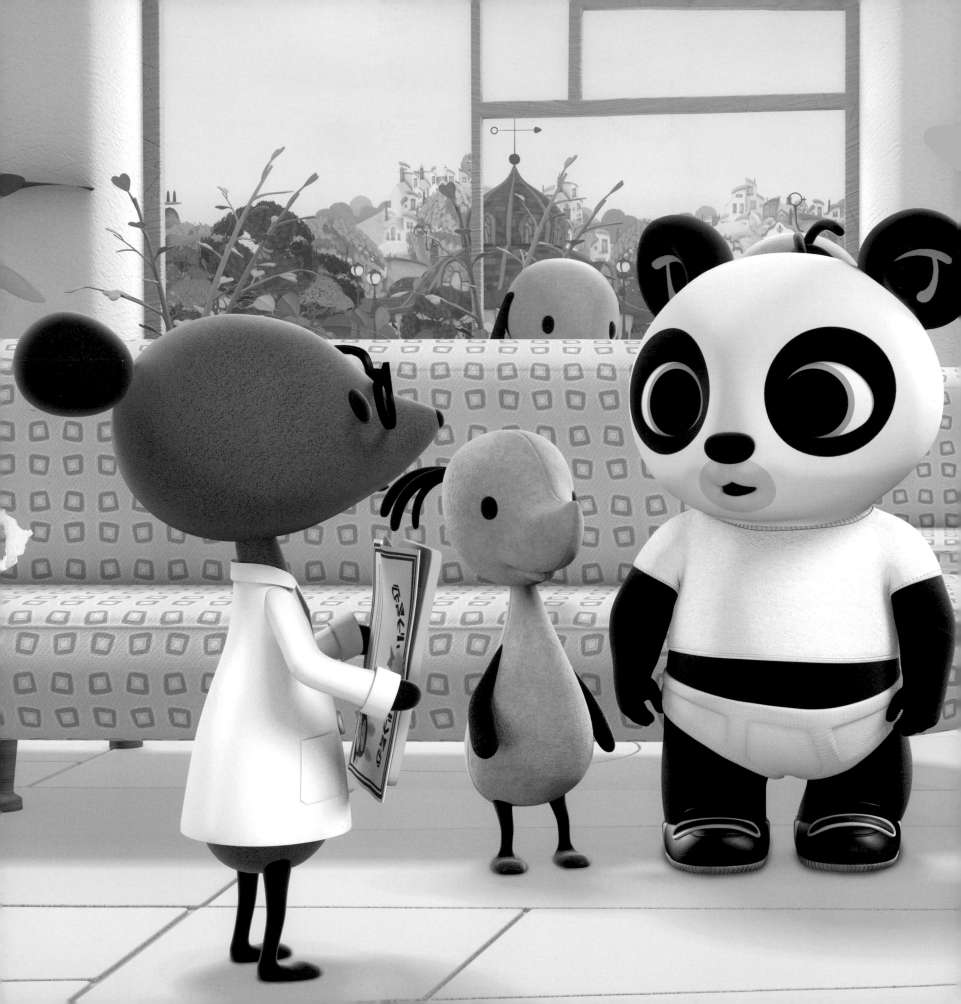

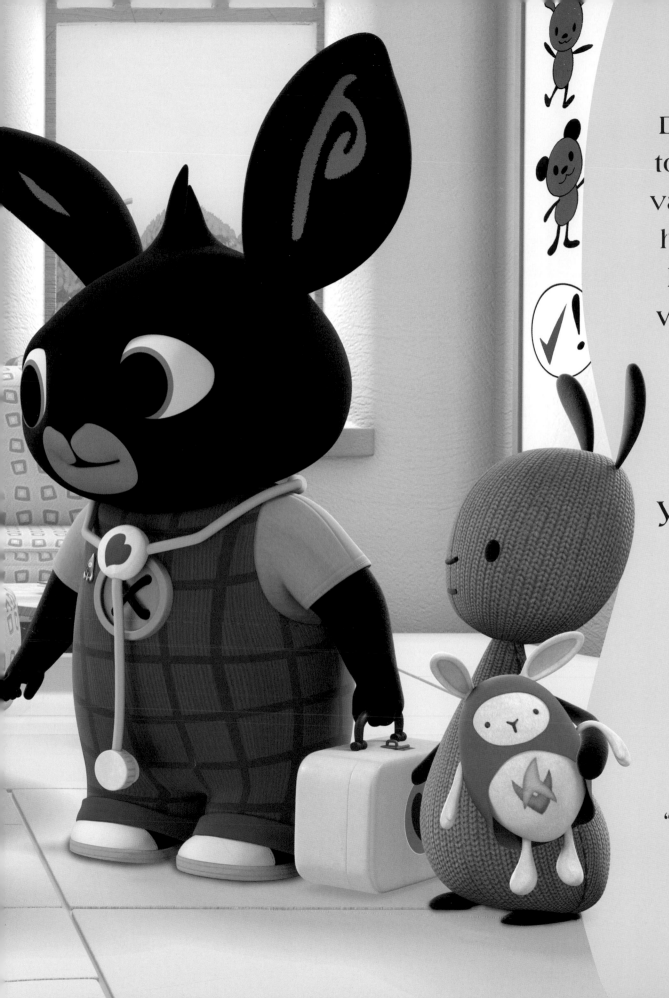

Dr Bing explains to Pando that the vaccination might hurt a teeny-tiny bit, but then he will get a sticker! Bing shows Pando his rocket one. **"Oh, I like your sticker!"** says Pando happily.

"Are you feeling ready now, Pando?" asks Dr Molly. "Yes, I think so," replies Pando.

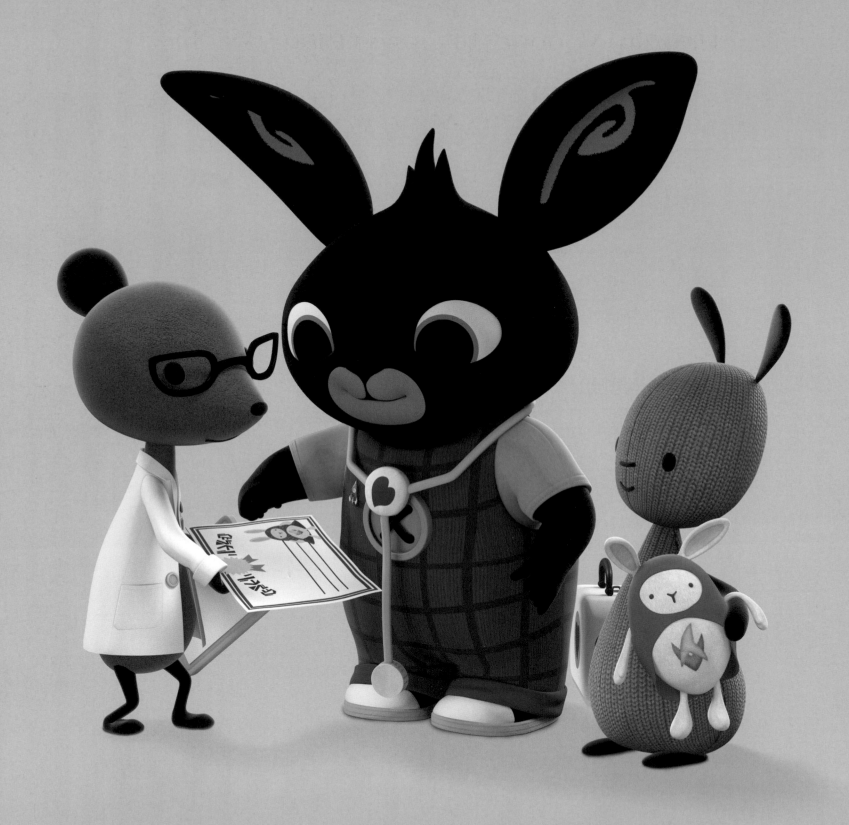

Dr Molly comes over to Bing. "I don't get many doctor
patients, so I almost forgot." She hands something special
to Bing. "It's a certificate to say how well you did."

"Hoppity Vooooosh!" gasps Bing, delighted.
"It's a Hoppity Voosh certificate!"
Bing hugs it tightly. "Oh! Thank you Dr Molly!"

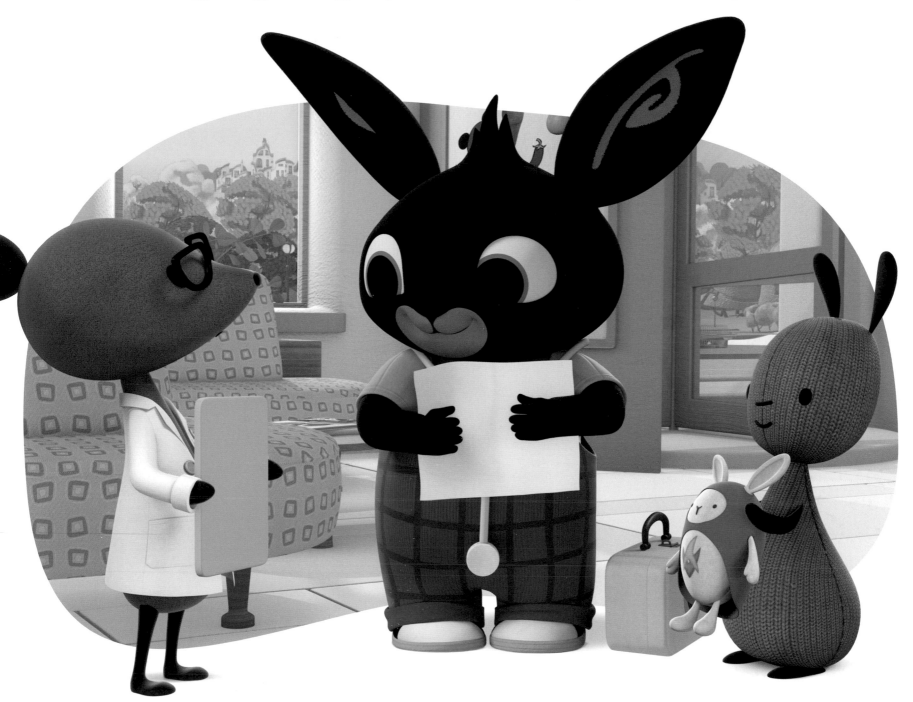

"No, thank *you*, Dr Bing!" says Dr Molly.
"Good for you, Bing!" says Flop.

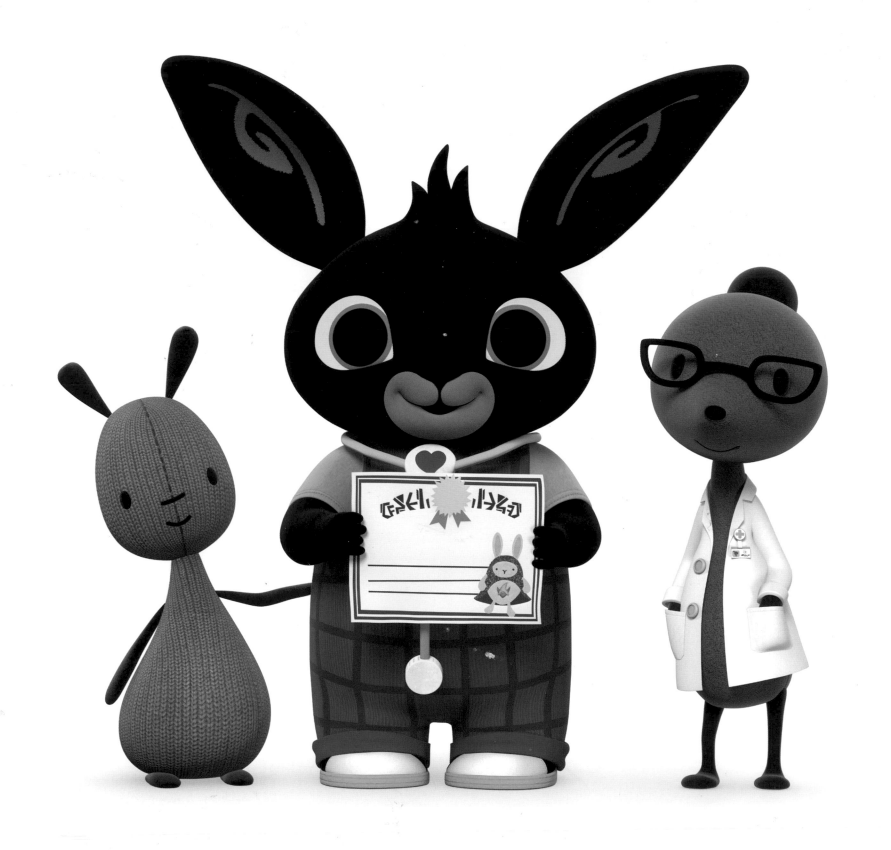

Going to the doctor . . . it's a Bing thing!